Back Pain
A Guide to Effective Back Pain Relief

By

Dermot Farrell

www.healbodymindandspirit.com

Copyright © 2017 and beyond Dermot Farrell

All Rights Reserved. No part of this publication may be reproduced in any form or by any means, including scanning, photocopying, or otherwise without prior written permission of the copyright holder.

Disclaimer and Terms of Use: The Author and Publisher has strived to be as accurate and complete as possible in the creation of this book, notwithstanding the fact that he does not warrant or represent at any time that the contents within are accurate due to the rapidly changing nature of the Internet. While all attempts have been made to verify information provided in this publication, the Author and Publisher assumes no responsibility for errors, omissions, or contrary interpretation of the subject matter herein. Any perceived slights of specific persons, peoples, or organizations are unintentional. In practical advice books, like anything else in life, there are no guarantees of income made. This book is not intended for use as a source of legal, business, accounting or financial advice. All readers are advised to seek services of competent professionals in legal, business, accounting, and finance field.

First Printing, 2017

MEDICAL DISCLAIMER

The information in this book is not intended to replace professional medical supervision. The information in this book is highly effective and it will definitely reduce and possible even reverse back pain symptoms in most individuals. In some cases a cure may take place; however, there is no guarantee that physical ailments will be completely cured. Prior to reducing or stopping allopathic medications, do consult with a qualified physician.

Contents

Introduction – Back Pain – Why do we have back pain and what to do about it	**7**
Chapter One – Types of Back Pain	**10**
Why Do We Get Back Pain?	12
Types of Back Pain	14
Chronic vs. Acute back Pain	14
Muscular Pain? Ligaments & Tendons/Nerves	15
Strains, Sprains. Ruptured (Herniated Discs)	16
Back Pain from a Traditional Chinese Medical (TCM) Perspective	19
Chapter Two – Getting the Basics Right!	**21**
Emotional Factors in Back Ache	23
General Good Advice for Back Pain Prevention and Rehab	24
Chapter Three – Acupressure Points for Back Pain Relief	**28**
Chapter Four – Myofascial Trigger Points	**35**
Part Two – Treating Back Pain	**40**
Chapter Five – Remedial Exercises for Back Pain	**41**

Spasms	42
Treating Back Pain with Remedial Exercises	43
Stretching to Relieve Back Pain	44
Stretching Guidelines	44
Stretching Exercises	45
Neck and Shoulders	45
Back Stretching	46
Hip and Glute Stretch	46
Hip and Glute Activation	47
Piriformis Muscle Stretch	48
Hamstring Stretching	49
Calf Stretches	50
McKenzie Exercises for Slipped or Herniated Discs	51
Core Strengthening Exercises	54
Uddiyana Bandha	55
Cat and Cow	55
The Plank	57
Back Strengthening Exercises	57
Resistance Exercises	58
Making Sense out of Remedial Back Exercises – Where to Start	61

Chapter Six – Hatha Yoga 63

Uttanasana (Intense Forward-Bending Pose)	66

Pashchimottanasana (Seated Forward Bend)	67
Bhujangasana (Cobra)	68
Adho mukha śvānāsana (downward-facing dog Pose)	70
Bālāsana (Child's Resting Pose)	72
ARDHA MATSYENDRASANA (Half Spinal Twist Pose)	73
Chapter Seven - Herbal Remedies for Back Pain	**75**
Herbal Teas for Back Pain Relief	75
Tumeric	75
Valerian Root	75
Eucommia	76
White Willow Bark	76
Devils Claw	76
Black Cohosh	76
Kava Kava	76
How to Make Herbal Tea	77
Free Gift	78

Introduction – Back Pain – Why do we have back pain and what to do about it

Do you suffer with back pain?

Is your quality of life impaired by back pain?

Do you get a bland and unhelpful response from most health professionals?

Do you feel like your aging too quickly and don't know what to do about it?

Well if you answered positively to most of these questions then you can regard yourself as quite normal, particularly if you are middle aged or elderly. The simple facts of life, for our backs, is that the human back was actually designed for qudrapedal movement, we are not really designed to be bipedal in the first place. Add in some wear and tear and age, a sedentary lifestyle and some age related degeneration and there you go back pain!

The nasty thing with back pain is that it's an icky kind of pain which either creeps up when we're not expecting it and suddenly we have chronic back pain whereby we can hardly move at all or it explodes out of nowhere, we get an acute bout of back pain and we can hardly lie down, sit down or even stand up!

Some years back I used to work in a job whereby I had to drive for many hours a day fairly frequently, as in two or three times a year I would suddenly get this acute back pain which would come from nowhere and last a good week or two before going away. I felt ok while sitting down, but sitting down or getting up became an absolute agony!

Back pain is usually not a very serious health condition and most doctors treat it in a lethargic kind of way with a few comments about looking after yourself and a prescription for some pain killers, but the simple reality, for anyone who regularly suffers with back ache, is that it is extremely debilitating!

Regarding my experience with treating back pain, I have a background in Traditional Chinese Medicine (TCM) and our stock and trade is treating back and shoulder problems much of the time, so I have seen my fair share of bad backs over the years. The good news from a TCM point of view, is that back pain is very treatable but the bad news is that there is a huge variety of causes and potential cure's for back ache. I myself have suffered on and off with a variety of back pain issues over the last few years and only recently I suffered quite a bit with lower back pain upon waking, only to find the condition suddenly clearing up all by itself practically overnight! So this is another issue with back aches, in that back ache can be an extremely painful ailment and often causes are hard to understand and a back ache can last month's only to suddenly disappear overnight!

The reason for this is because of the complexity of the muscles in the back and how they relate to each other. We shall take a look at these in us a chapter one, but for now what can we say about back ache and what can this book do to help you?

As far as I am concerned nothing makes you feel old like back ache does, whereby you end up walking like one of those mummies from those old black and white movies. Having difficulty sitting, standing, walking and lying down or even moving immediately makes you feel old and question your own youthfulness. The thought "is this it is I now grown old?" often passes through most people's minds when they feel like this. Also back ache does not respect youth either, while most people who suffer a lot with back ache will do so from their 30's /40's upwards, there are lots of young people who also become afflicted with back pain at an early age!

Regarding this book and what it can do for your back pain, it can certainly help a lot but to what degree I can to tell you. My experience with back ache over the years has lead me to believe that back ache is usually a symptom of postural imbalances and can be straightened out surprisingly quickly, once you get a handle on it. So this is the good news. But the bad news is that there are lots of variations in back ache, causes and treatments, plus as we age we develop more long-term degeneration which is not curable. So in a nutshell in some cases back pain can be completely cured, whereas in others it can simply be greatly improved. But certainly if you follow the advice in this book, you will find yourself getting back pain less frequently and the bouts of back pain will be far less intense and will last for a shorter period of time!

To some degree we all have to live with our backs, which are a complex arrangement of joints, ligaments, tendons and muscles and also to some degree we can really improve and even cure our aching backs, in a far shorter time than we may realise. So get reading and start applying these back relieving strategies today!

Chapter One – Types of Back Pain

In order to understand the different types of back pain, we have to begin by taking a look at a diagram of our backs.

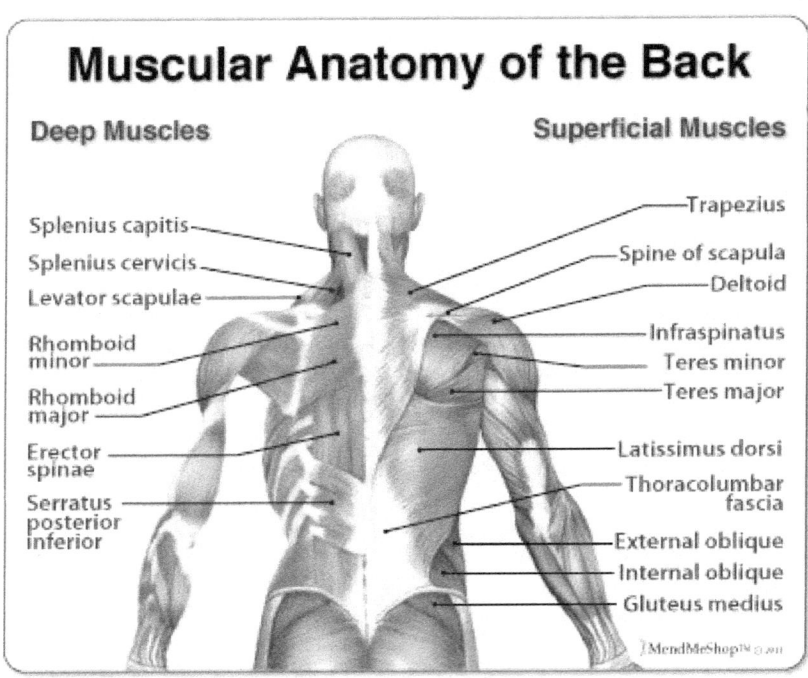

Ok if we take a look at this diagram, we see a total of 18 muscles listed (although only 16 of them are back muscles, as the deltoid is the shoulder muscle and the gluteus maximus is the ass muscle). If we simplify it a little bit we find out that the following major groups have a big effect on back health:

Spinor Erectors – These are the two pillars like muscle groups which run from the base of the spine up to the first quarter of your back. These are the sort of muscles which often give out suddenly when we overload the lower back.

Latissimus Dorsi - These are the wing like muscles on either side of the torso, which can flare out in the case of athletes. They are the second biggest group of muscles in the back and are quite prone to getting pulled resulting sometimes as a chronic pain and sometimes as an acute pain.

Trapezius-Is a huge muscle which runs from the mid back all the way up to the neck. This is the muscle which when well-developed gives the appearance of a hump at the lower part of the neck. The trapezius are used to shrug and pull the back upwards and often flare ups can occur here.

Other Muscle Groups - Other popular muscles groups for getting hurt are the rhomboids, teres major and minor muscles of the mid and upper back and also the muscles on the side of the neck which re the splenius capitis and the splenius cervicis muscles.

Joint Damage –Although you cannot see it in this picture, the back is built upon the spine which is a large bony structure which consists of several sections, including the lower lumber region, the main thoracic region and also the ones of the neck itself. With age comes some degeneration, also lifting heavy weights with bad posture, sedentary living a lack of physical balance can all put pressure on resulting in imbalances in the spine. The most common damage here tend to either be ruptured or prolapsed discs, which are the jelly like liquid sandwich, which allows one spinal joint to rest upon another and usually this occur in the lower lumber region near the spinor rector muscles. Also due to bad posture often some damage can occur to the bones in the neck as well. And of course blunt trauma, such as falling and car accidents will often damage the spine to some degree.

Why Do We Get Back Pain?

The reasons for back pain are quite varied, the simplest answer been that we are not really designed to walk on two legs and that our backs lack the structural integrity to hold this weight well. If you add in poor posture, lack of exercise and sometimes blunt trauma into the equation, we can easily see how back pain can develop and indeed by middle age most people have some degree of off and on bouts of back pain!

Regarding the region of the back which suffers with pain, often the part of the back which is feeling sore is not actually the cause of the pain.

Often where the pain originates is not where the pain is from in the first place!

Ok let's get this straight, say for instance you are suffering with a chronic pain on your lower left side near your left spinor erectors, chances are that the cause is actually on the right hand side of the body, possibly the right lower back although, it doesn't have to be, as it could be originating from another area of the right side of the back altogether!

So what's happening here is that the right side is suffering with a postural imbalance, due to a sedentary lifestyle, or possibly blunt trauma and for a while the left side picks up the slack, then one fine day the left hand side cannot take it anymore and suddenly we get either a stabbing pain in the left hand side, or if this is a recurrent type of pain we simply get that old dull ache which we have suffered from before. The tendency is to think that the left hand side is the cause and it is the cause in the sense that this muscle is now damaged and needs to repair itself, but the actual cause began with the rightandside and the left had side adapted for a while before it suddenly blew out!

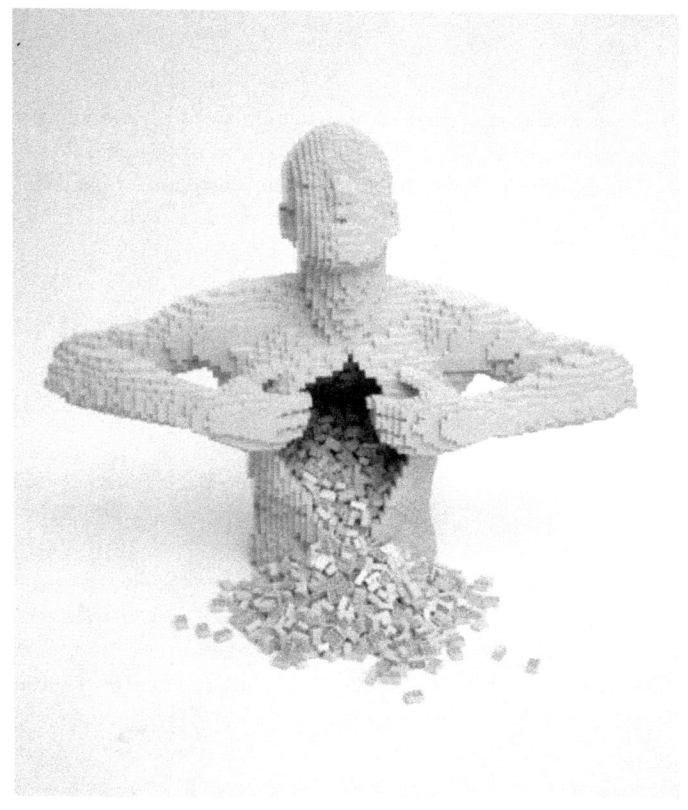

In many ways the back can be liked to a stack of Lego's, whereby each Lego seats upon another Lego and all is well until one or two of the Legos are pulled out and the entire stack of Lego's comes falling down. So it's easy when we see muscular diagrams to think that each of these muscle groups simply doing its thing, when in fact they are all interrelated. So every time we pull our back out, one area of the back stops working properly and other areas chip in to bear the load, until finally one gives away. Really it's quite an amazing adapatative system in the human body, whereby we can rapidly adapt to muscular imbalances. But also this explains why yesterday we had a pain in our left lower side, today we have a pain in our mid upper back and tomorrow we end up having a pain in our upper right hand side!

It's extremely common and quite irritating as it's hard to know what to do about it. In the next chapter, we will start to go into more detail about how we can treat back pain effectively, but briefly we shall take a look at the different types of aches and pains, in order to better understand the nature of the health condition which we want to treat.

Types of Back Pain

Chronic vs. Acute back Pain

Firs to all let's get our head around the difference between chronic and acute back pain. Acute means that the pain is sudden and sharp in nature, while chronic usually entails a dull repetitive, but less severe ache. But to some degree this can be misleading, for often we get a sudden new pain and it's acute, it came from nowhere and it hurts like hell but, what are we supposed to about it? Finally we make some progress and also nature heals us over a period of time, then the acute pain disappears and is replaced by a dull pain which lasts for a longer period of time, so this pain can be viewed as chronic. Also usually when the pain comes back again it will be a chronic pain, as in it will be a dull pain, although in some cases it will come back as an acute pain!

So we can't really easily distinguish between chronic and acute, save to say that if the pain is intense and the onset is sudden then it's acute, whereas a dull ache which lingers around and then kicks in from time it time is seen to be a chronic pain.

Muscular Pain? Ligaments & Tendons/Nerves

Muscular pain is a pain which originates in any of the major muscles groups listed earlier. As for ligaments and tendons, these are connective tissues which connect the muscles to the bones and points and help the body to move. The cause of pain in either muscles or ligaments and tendons is often very similar, but usually damage to a ligament or tendon will take a long time to cure.

The famous Achilles heel tendon is a tendon which attaches to the back of the heel and athletes, in particular, football players are prone to damaging this tendon which often results in many months of rehabilitation. Tendons and ligaments are damaged less frequently than muscles which are a good thing as they take a long time to heal and often even then sometimes a fair degree of damage still persists. Also with tendons it is a very easy thing to develop tendonitis of any tendon, which is over worked due to repetitive action. For this reason tendonitis often occurs in the wrists and elbows, which are hardworking joints, but also we can develop some degree of either tendonitis or general tendon inflammation, in our lower backs, if we overdo it through either sport or exercise, so be careful about any kind of repetitive action. For example, say you're in a job whereby you have to keep turning to one side and moving items, say for example working on the check out in a supermarket, whereby you have to move many items on your left side only or on your right, this repetitive movement could cause either muscle soreness or in some case even inflammation of the tendons in the lower back. I know it sounds silly, but silly bad habits if repeated often enough will cause damage and damage will result in pain!

Nerve damage of course is in a separate class all of its own. With nerve damage usually a nerve has got caught, more often not in a joint and this impinges upon the nerve. This can result in pain and irritation and in some case nerve damage is permanent. The most famous type of nerve damage affecting the back is sciatic, whereby the nerve running from the leg up to the hip gets impinged, often sudden sparking lights are seen in the eyes and it comes on with a sudden extremely sharp pain and ends up taking anywhere from days to weeks to recover from. Other less famous but equally irritating areas, for never pain, are in the shoulders and neck and can often result either from blunt trauma like an accident or as a consequence of bad postural habits.

Strains, Sprains. Ruptured (Herniated Discs)

A strain occurs when we put too much load on a muscle, tendon or ligament over time. A good example would be working in the garden and developing an achy back after a few hours of heavy lifting and bending over for long periods of time, resulting in the back getting slightly strained and developing a lower back ache. Also sometimes if you bend over for a long time, when you go to stand up instead of developing a lower back ache you might end up with a sudden mid back ache which is quite sharp. In this case you have just sprained either your rhomboids or trapezius muscles!

So strains are a dull ache caused by overwhelming the muscle over a period of time, whereas sprains are sudden and sharp and usually come about a result of blunt trauma, falling of your bike for example. But then how can a person standing up after a long team of bending over sprain their upper back, where is the blunt trauma here? What's happened here is that the back probably already has some issues whereby some muscles in the upper back are getting stained and so others are over working, then when you go to stand up the various upper back muscles operate and as they do so the weakest link in the chain suddenly snaps and we get a sprain!

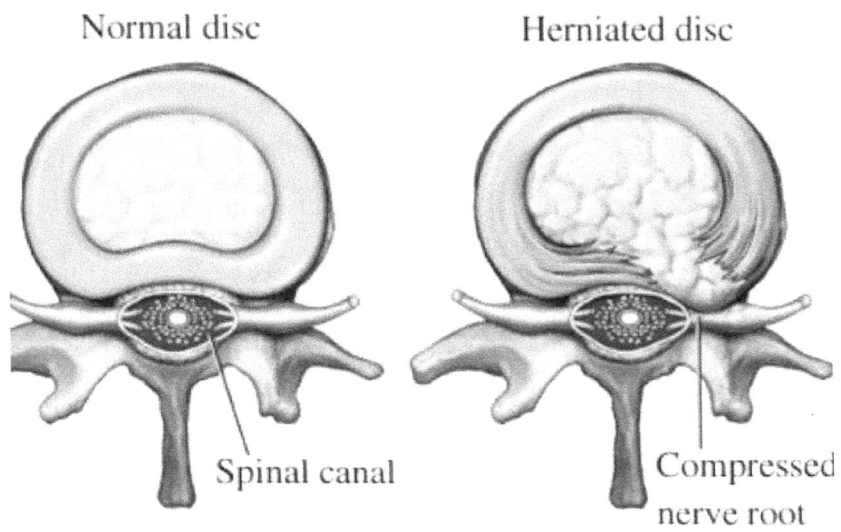

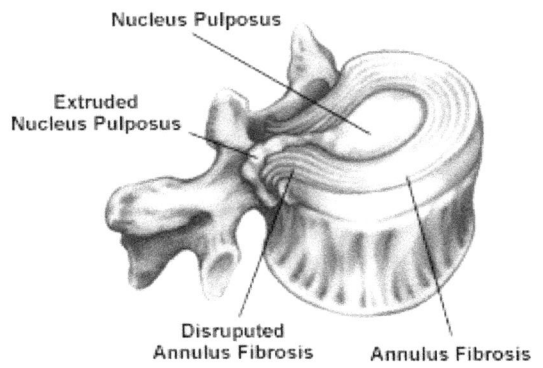

Rupture (herniated) discs are of course a much more severe problem. The disc acts like cushions which seepage each of the vertebrae (spinal joints, there are 33 vertebrae in total (7 in the neck, 12 in the thoracic region, 5 in the lobar region, 5 in the sacral region and 3 in the coccygeal region)).With age they can dry out and expand slightly beyond the width of the vertebrae, thus giving the appearance of a burger coming out between two burger buns. However, sometimes some of the nucleus pulposus extrudes, thus created a herniated (protruding) or ruptured disc, as it is sometimes called.

Treating the herniated disc is difficult and also it can be extremely painful. In some cases medical operations are required and usually once a disc ruptures it becomes a lifelong problem.

There is no simple strategy for treating a herniated disc, although everything mentioned in this book will help. If you suffer with a herniated disc it is well worth your while visiting with an acupuncturist as in many clinical trials they noted an actual improvement in the disc health, after an extensive bout of acupuncture. Acupuncture is the only treatment which I am aware of which has been clinically proven to heal herniated discs, in some cases. Although to achieve this will usually take many months of acupuncture!

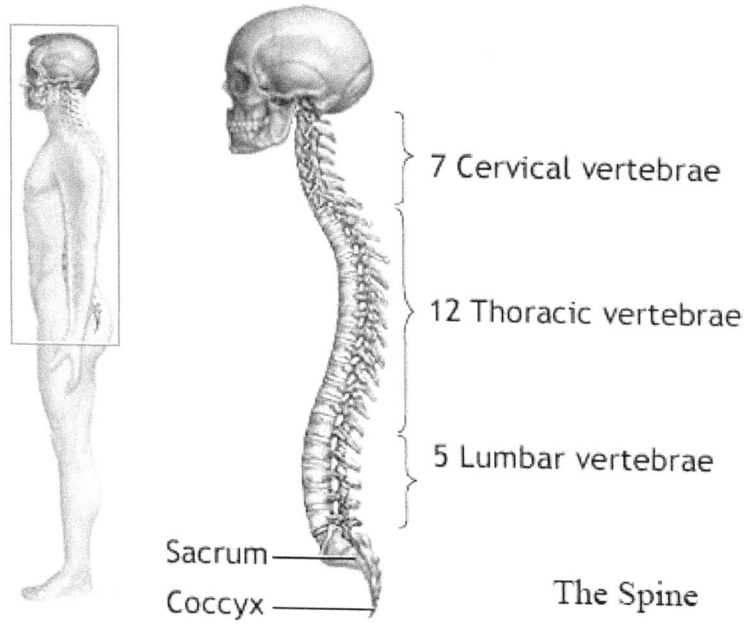

Back Pain from a Traditional Chinese Medical (TCM) Perspective

From a TCM perspective all back pain originates from an energetic imbalance. In Chinese medicine the focus is on Qi (pronounced as Chi) energy and it is divided into yang Qi (active energy) and Ying Qi (nurturing energy). Also these energies run along energetic lines of force throughout the body, which are known as meridians.

Now there's all sorts of reasons as to why we get back pain from a TCM point of view, but put very briefly we tend to get back pain either because energy is deficient somewhere or because it is stagnant (not moving), both of which will eventually result in an excess of energy on one of the channels which will realty in a strain or a sprain in our back muscles.

The question then is how can this knowledge help us to repair this damage?

Well the great thing about TCM is that it demonstrates how our back pain is caused by energetic imbalances and if we correct these imbalances we will correct our bad backs too. From an allopathic point of view, it can be all too easy to see back pain as a mixture of bad lifestyle and posture, but when we delve more deeply via Chinese medicine, we discover that our painful backs have usually kicked off because they are weak backs in the first place, as a consequence of energetic imbalances.

From a treatment point of view TCM and in particular acupuncture can be a very helpful therapy to apply when you have severe back ache, but even if you don't go to an acupuncturist take this message away, which is that the achy back is an energetically imbalanced back. Consequently we have to look at lifestyle, diet and even overall health and wellbeing levels, if we want to cure our back ache!

Chapter Two – Getting the Basics Right!

In chapter two we looked at length at the various causes of back ache. At the very end we looked at what Traditional Chinese Medicine (TCM) had to say about back ache, which is that back ache comes from an energetic imbalance, which is usually either a deficiency or a stagnating of energy. Now in part two of this book we shall look at detail at the various self-treatment options which are available to you, but prior to doing this in this chapter we are going to take a quick look at getting the basics right!

There is a tendency to think that a bad back has come about because of some misfortune, genetic predisposition or blunt trauma, and while this might all be true, we have to look a little deeper than this if we want to resolve our back ache issues.

On a deeper level the following factors have a strong predetermining effect on back pain:

- Genetics
- Lifestyle
- Accidents
- Diet
- Stress levels
- Nurture
- Balance

The first three are very obvious. Some of us are genetically predetermined towards having back aches and in particular people with long backs tend to develop more back problems than people will shorter backs, as the leverage of the back which is entirely genetically predetermined, can have a big effect on back aches. Lifestyle of course is a big factor, and in particular a sedentary lifestyle will result in muscular imbalances and also a weakening of the muscles of the back, core and stomach area, making the body more prone to back aches. Finally, accidents can happen at any time and they do affect the back in a very negative manner, as often blunt trauma exerts itself on the trunk of the body, which in turn sprains or even tears the muscles of the back.

So this is the obvious stuff, but what is not so obvious is that our diet can affect our backs because if our diet is un-nutritious it will weaken Qi, which will make us more prone to having a weak back, which in turn will make straining our backs more likely to happen.

Stress levels are also important as one of the energy meridians (the liver meridian) controls the smooth flow of energy throughout the body, so when we get angry and frustrated our energy through the body gets restricted, resulting either in a deficiency or a stagnation of liver Qi energy, which in turn throws of other energetic changes (most likely the bladder channel in the case of the back). So when we are stressed, it opens up our bodies to a plethora of complaints which includes back ache.

How nurtured we are as people also has an effect. In Chinese medicine our ying energy is our nurturing energy and if we feel deflated, unloved, put upon and generally not appreciated it can also undermine the back in the same way as the liver stagnation or deficiency, in that our ying becomes weak which in turn affects the yang/yang energetic imbalance.

How balanced is our life is another important point, for when our lives are out of balance it once again disrupts the yang/yang balance which in turn can result in back ache.

Emotional Factors in Back Ache

The human body is an amazing construct and when we apply the principles of Traditional Chinese Medicine to it, we can see that having an achy back is as much an energetic imbalance as it is a physical one!

But we can take it a step further. We find that the body is a symbolic representation of the mind. Now this might sound a bit irregular, but to think of it this way, take a look at the cars and trucks on the road and you shall notice that they all have two head lights and a grill, if you look carefully you will see that they look like a face, with the headlights been eyes and the grill been the mouth!

The reason for this is that unconsciously we all think in a symbolic way, without realising it we can project our vision of ourselves onto the world around us. This doesn't just apply to the world around us as it also applies to our own bodies as well.

If we think about the back, we have phrases like "education is the backbone of society" and "person x is the backbone of this family", for example. Why do we do this? We do this because it's a metaphor representing our feelings that just like how the backbone supports the body, so too does a certain societal organisation or family member support either society itself or the family as a whole. But if we think about it, often when we have back pain, the back pain represents some imbalance in our own lives. If our back is stiff, for example, maybe in some way we could be more adaptable in our own lives. If we have a posture problem and can't stand up straight, maybe we feel weighed down by some worry or concern. Also if we have a nagging pain in one part of our back maybe we have some inner insecurity problem at work here.

I'm not suggesting that every back ache has some unconscious emotional motivation behind it, but if you do all the right things and still keep on getting reoccurring back problems, maybe there is some unconscious stress or concern, which is making you more prone to back ache in the first place!

I'm not trying to over mystify the subject, but in many cases there is a mental emotional element in curing back ache. Especially when we think in terms of our backs holding our bodies up. Without our back, we would not be able to stand or move around, so it is only natural that when we have some mental or emotional stressors in our live, that they would affect the part of our body which represents this same quality.

So if you are having back problems and have tried out everything under the sun, then try and think in terms of stress, mental and emotional triggers, which might be releasing themselves under the guide of back pain, it's worth a try!

General Good Advice for Back Pain Prevention and Rehab

Before moving onto part two, where we shall go into depth regarding the various strategies for easing back pain, let's take a quick look first at some basic good advice, chances are you already heard this before, but then again it's always a good idea to reiterate good advice.

If you go to your general practitioner/family doctor, chances are that they will ask you about lifestyle and that they will suggest that you eat healthy, get out and exercises and try to de-stress and basically they are right to say this.

Diet is very important, as noted earlier a poor diet can result in energetic imbalances, which can make us more prone to developing ill health. But also even away from purely nutritional point of view it makes sense to eat a healthy diet, so as to provide the body with whatever it requires for growth and repair. Also there are some unique considerations. Young people and kids need to get in a lot of calcium, as their bones are young and developing and also menopausal women often lack calcium so once again it's a good idea to take some calcium and vitamin D has to be imbibed at the same time, for the body to process it properly.

If we take the example of menopausal women and post menpsapusl women, often their bones are weak from a lack of calcium and the lack of oestrogen hormone, has an effect too in reducing bone strength. Osteoporosis is a common disease in the elderly and particular amongst women. Taking some calcium supplementation is a good idea, so as to maintain the integrity of the bones of the spine, ribcage and neck.

Furthermore exercises are important. From appaorximatley 50 years of age on a condition called as sarcopenia sets in. Sarcopenia is age related muscular wastage and it occurs in both men and women and even in athletic types and weight lifters some degree of sarcopenia will set in. After the age of 50, the average person will lose anywhere between 0.5–1% of muscle loss per year!

So by the time a person has reached 70, there's a good chance that they will have lost possible 20 to 30% of their muscle mass!

Now this might not sound interesting, especially if you're not into sports or weight training, but the simple reality is that nobody can afford to lose 10%+ of their lean muscle mass per decade, over the age of 50. It's this wasting away of muscle which makes a lot of people weak and fragile, by the time they get into their late 60's or early 70's. While it's impossible to prevent sarcopenia from taking place, it can be reduced to a great degree by living an active lifestyle. The best policy is to go to the gym and workout with weights for three times a week. If that sounds daunting, then at least get active, try and do some rigorous exercises like swimming or squash or tennis and if you cannot do these activities then at least go for a walk. By supporting our musculature we are supporting good posture, which in turn will both rehab old injuries to our backs and prevent future injured from taking place!

In particular we need to get active. Our modern lifestyle is very sedentary; most of us end up just sitting around. The problem with just sitting around is that we get muscle wastage (even if we're young), simply because we do not move our muscles. Secondly our hip abductors become tight, which in turn results in tightness of the lower back and stiffness of the hips and even knee joints. Also sitting with our heads slumped over our keyboard plays havoc with the subtle structure of our upper thoracic vertebrae (vertebrae of the upper trunk) and our neck vertebrae. Plus it restricts breathing, which in turn makes us less energetic and less healthy.

So before you read another page of this book take a quick assessment.

Are you eating well?

Are you resting well?

Are you exercising regularly?

Do you go to the gym, play sports or at east go for a walk every day?

If you can answer yes to most of these questions then move on top part two, where we will look at a wide variety of exercises and treatments which can help your back health, if not then take a look at your lifestyle, for no matter what treatment you try, unless you get the basics right you will keep on having bouts of back pain. Often when we get frequent bouts of an ache in or body, it's our body's way of telling us something so that we can make changes and improve things. Don't hide away from any hints from your body, listen up and make whatever changes need to be made so as to assure long-term back health!

Chapter Three – Acupressure Points for Back Pain Relief

Acupuncture is well known for its efficacy in treating back pain and if you are suffering with a lot of back pain problems it might be one of the therapies which you should consider trying out by visiting with an acupuncturist. If you take a look at the diagram below you will see just how many acupuncture points run along the length of your back, so when you go to an acupuncturist they will put needles in these 'local' points, plus they will also use some distant points, which are referred to as 'distal' points, for example one such point is on the back of your knee, another is near the ankle, another is on your hand and another on your wrist. So it might feel unusual but it can work wonders.

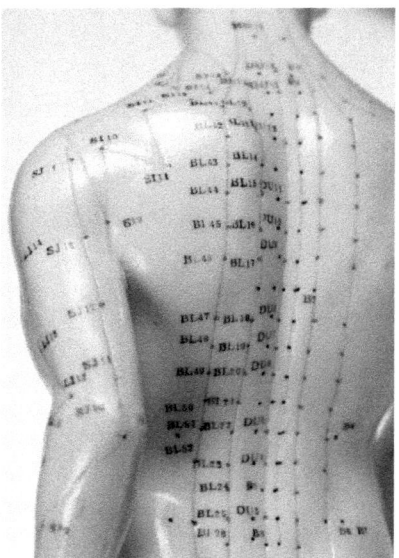

However, what if you don't want to visit an acupuncturist or even you do visit with an acupuncturist or some other complementary therapist once or twice a week, but you want to do something on a daily basis to help you?

This is where acupressure comes in. Acupressure works upon the same principles as acupuncture but its application is a little less effective, as no needles are involved. However it still works the same meridians, thus helping to boost deficiencies, move stagnant energy and reduce excessive energy in the channels.

The acupressure points which follow are very easy to apply and all you have to do is to find the point and then apply a good bit of pressure for a few minutes or so. What most people do wrong with acupressure, is they take a namby pamby approach, whereby they hardly touch the point. This is the wrong approach, rather you must find the point and exert considerable pressure to the point that it aches a little bit, when you get that achy feeling going on, then hold that point for at least two or three minutes.

Now this can become really tiring on your fingers, so you can use acupressure point pressure tools or simply use the blunt end of a pen or pencil of you have to. If you have a pen with a pointy lid, you can start by applying dull pressure with the flat end of the open and then to take it up a gear after a couple of minutes by applying the pointy head, which is a sharper point, it will ache more but also it will heighten the effectiveness.

You can use acupressure as often as you like, ideally twice a day when you have a back ache is good, although you could carry out another extra session if you have to go out somewhere and want some relief before you go out!

Ling Gui & Da Bai

These are two acupuncture points which can also be used with acupressure. If you take a look at the picture below, these two points run along the bone of the hand. Now the idea with these two points if you arch your hand as is seen in this picture, you will see the bone of your hand as representing your spine, with one difference it's in inverse. So Ling Gui represents the lower back and Da Bai represents the upper back.

How to work these points, simply apply pressure back and forth along this line and whenever you feel tenderness focus your efforts there.

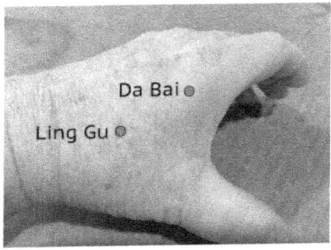

Picture courtesy of www.catstcmnotes.com

Gallbladder 34

Gallbladder 34 is a point which is found on the lateral (outside) aspect of the leg, and is just in front of the bony outer part of the calf bone (head of the fibula) and slightly higher than it. To locate this point find the bony outer edge of your knee and lower your finger until it touches the bony head of the femur. Now move your finger forward ahead of the bony head and slightly upwards of it. I know this might be as clear as mud, but just poke around and after a while when you find a tender spot just start pressing it. Gallbladder 34 when combined with Ling Gui and Da Bai is quite an effective way to treat lower back ache.

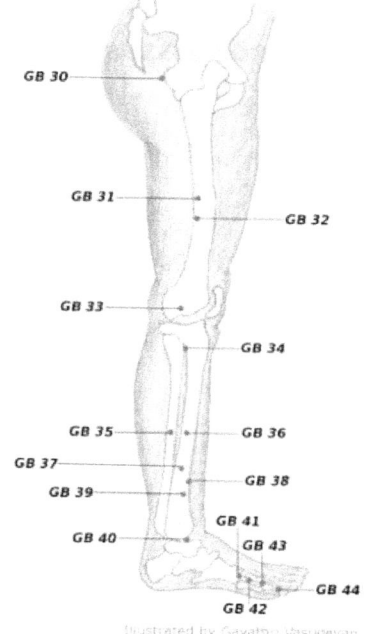

Gallbladder 36

Gallbladder 36 is located just above the knee cap directly parallel to gallbladder 34. To locate this point take your finger and feel the outer edge of your knee and then slide your finger upwards until it falls from the knee onto the outer thigh muscle, that's it. To double check give these areas a good squeeze and you will find a tender spot which is GB36. When combined with the other points above it is quite effective at treating back pain.

Small Intestine 4

Small intestine 4 is located on the outer side of your hand near your knuckles. To locate this point clench your fist and where the skin bulges outwards slightly this is si4. Simply press on this point with a sharpish point and it will give instant back relief.

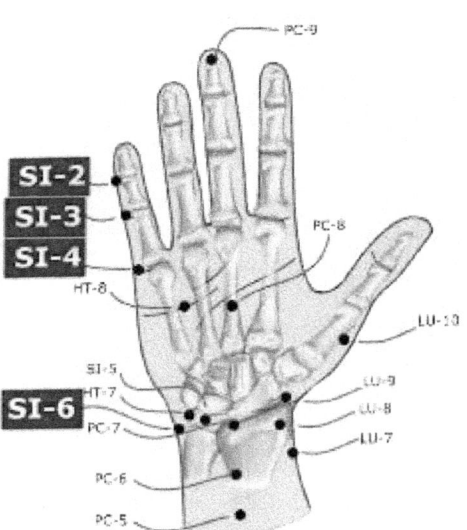

Bladder 40

Is located in the fleshy mass just behind the knee. Atypically in acupuncture we get the patient to lie down and then stick a needle deep into this point, although you can also needle from a standing position, but for acupressure you're going to have to get someone to come behind you and deep pressure message this point. So once again to locate it, stand up and feel the muscle behind your knee and right in the middle press deeply. The ideal approach with this point is to lift and thrust the needle so as to stimulate the bladder channel. Even with acupressure you can take the same approach by thrusting with your finger, acupressure device or pen and then letting go and then doing this repeatedly, press real hard then relax and back and forth so as to simulate this channel.

Bladder 57

Bladder 57 is located where the two side of the calf come together. Simple apply pressure to this point and relieve will come quickly.

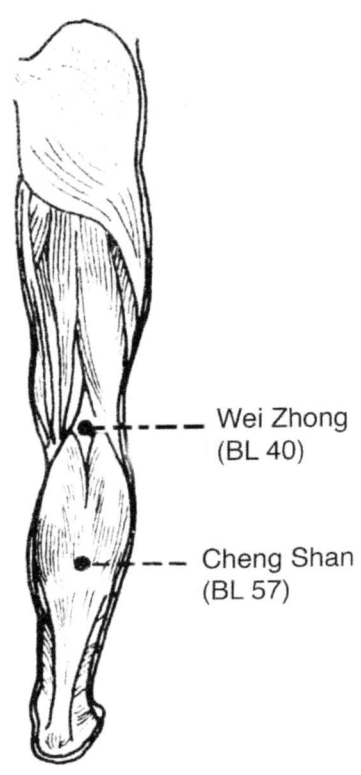

Chapter Four – Myofascial Trigger Points

Myofascial trigger points are points along the fascia (the flesh will holds the various muscles and organs in place), which when massaged deeply they release tension and pain. Often pain will travel along the fascia, so you might for example, have a pain in your left lower back, but when you massage your right buttock it releases the tension and the pain. Mysofacscial trigger points are quite an amazing way of releasing built up tension and trauma with in the fascia.

The fascia is elastic like substance which surrounds our muscles and organs and keeps everything in place. Think of it this way, why doesn't your stomach get displaced when you do a somersault?

Because it is held in place by the fascia!

Another example of fascia, which I think everyone can understand, is calf pain. Have you ever put your calves through a rigorous workout, maybe you over worked them in the gym, or possibly you went for a 10 mile hike up the side of a mountain. Either way you wake up the next day with a horrible pain in your calf' and moving was just agony. The reason for this is that the fascia surrounding your calf muscles is very tight and once the muscles expand rapidly, as a result of strenuous activity, it puts a huge amount of tension on the fascia and in turn it results in a lot of pain!

Regarding how to apply mysofascial massage, you can simply go for deep pressure with your fingers if you like, but also you can use various massage aids, out of which a cricket ball or tennis ball are probably the easiest one's which you can use!

Say, for example you feel pain in your lower back; you can simply stand in front of a wall and place the tennis ball or cricket ball directly behind where you feel pain and then press hard with your back thus squeezing the ball between your back and the wall. Now once you do this simply move up, down, left and right and keep on gyrating , putting on more pressure, then less and so on and just try and feel the pain and keep pressing and feeling the relieve as you do so. You can also do this with your neck, for example, if you have neck pain and of course you can press with your buttocks too!

Here are a couple of pictures which will outline some of the good myofascial trigger points which you can use to relieve your back ache:

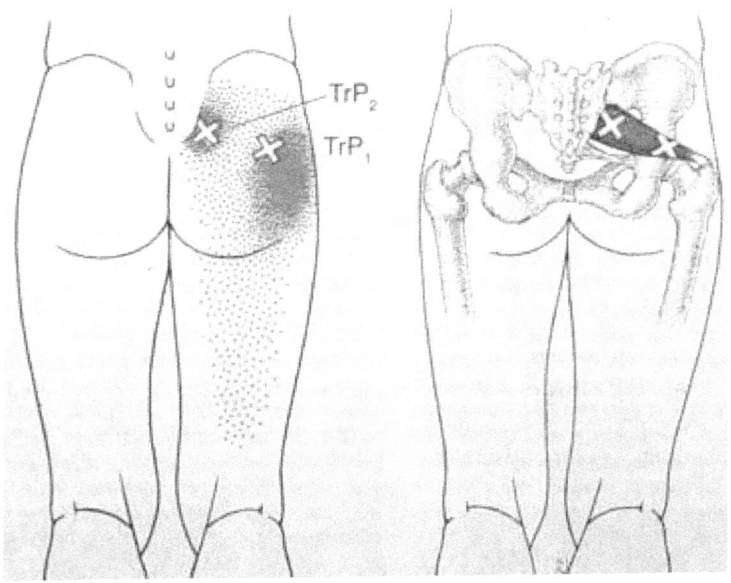

Piriformis

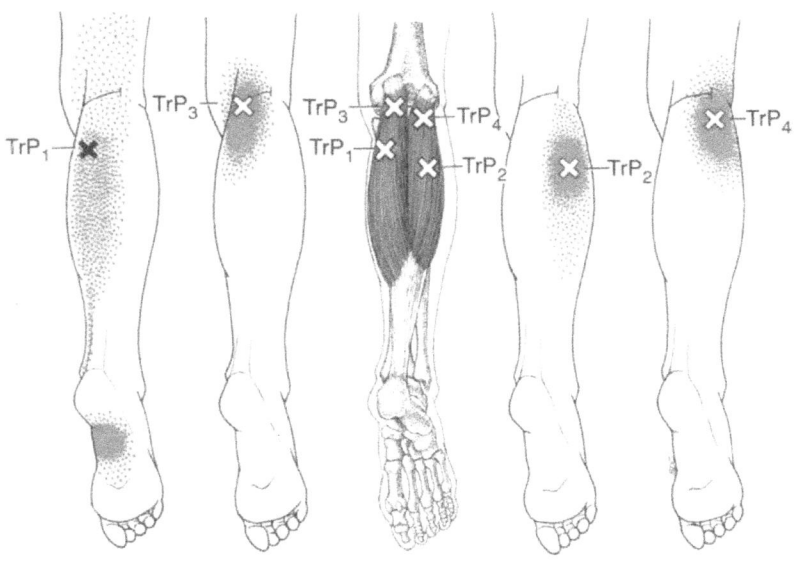

Soleus and Gastronemius

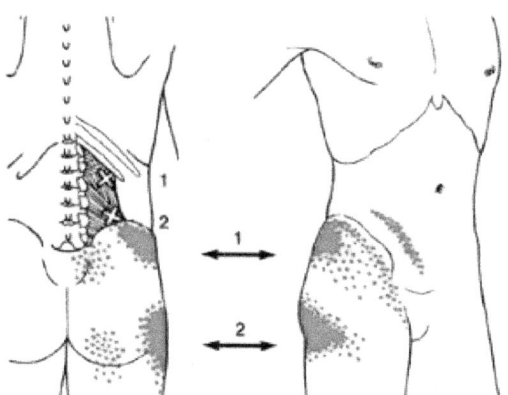

Quadratus Lumborum

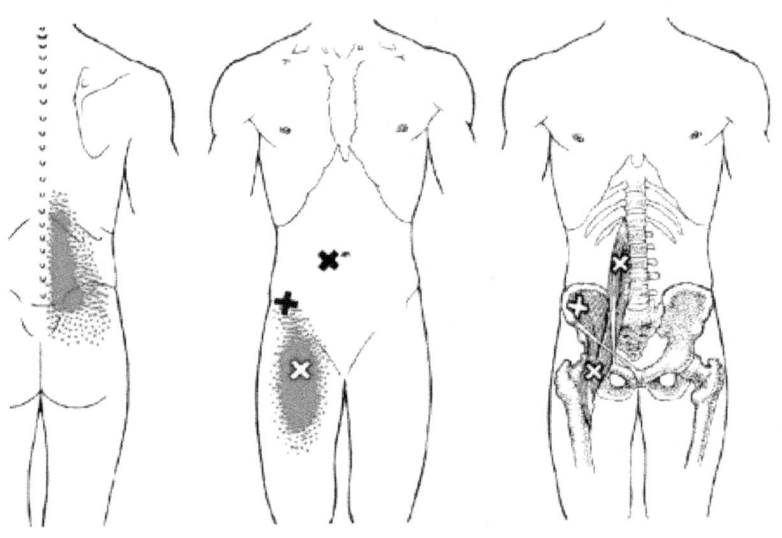

Iliopsoas

It's difficult to explain how best to work on these points without talking at great length. If you would like to pursue myofascial trigger point therapy in greater detail than check out my book on Trigger Point Therapy as it will go into lots of detail on how best to use trigger points to release not just back pain but pain in general through the body!

The best tip which I can give you for now is to take out a tennis ball or baseball or whatever so long as it's a fairly hard ball and find the area of pain and just massage your body by pressing this ball between your body and the wall or your body and the floor. It's really quite amazing. Sometimes I get lower back ache and I can usually cure it with less than a minute, by either pressing with my lower back against a cricket ball or taking the ball and placing it against my bottom and pressing it around this the area which lies between the hip bones and the buttock muscles (Gluteus maximus). This area is labelled as the Quadratus Lumborum (lower back) and the Iliopsoas (in the bottom near the hip). So a little bit of manipulation in this area can work wonders for lower back pain.

What about upper back pain and neck pain?

Well simply use the ball against the lattissimus dorsi or the romboids and trapezius muscles, for upper back and for neck pain simply take the ball and place it between your neck and either the wall or the floor (if you're lying down) and gently massage. Also for shoulder aches, either front or rear once again place the ball between your shoulder and the wall and press back and forth!

Part Two – Treating Back Pain

Chapter Five – Remedial Exercises for Back Pain

In the following chapters we shall look at a variety of approaches towards treating back pain, both from a rehabilitation point of view (rehab) and a preventative point of view (prehab). If you are prone to back ache then, these are good chapters to look at. However, what if you're in pain right now and want relief from back pain right now what should you do?

Well this is where this chapter can help. In this chapter we shall cover the main points regarding rehabilitating your back, before moving onto other longer term back health strategies in the subsequent chapters.

If we take a look at our backs there are three major muscle groups which we have to keep in mind if we want to rehab our backs, they are:

- **Extensors in the back and bottom (gluteal) muscles** – whose function is to straighten the back, so as to help us either stand or sit upright, lift objects, extend our body's outward and move our thighs away from our body's.

- **Flexors of the abdominal and iliopsoas muscles** – Whose function is to bend and support the spine from the front and also they help to control the arching of the lower (lumbar) spine, plus they help with moving the thighs towards our body's.

- **Oblique's which are also known as Rotators -** Are side muscles which help us to stabilize the spine when we are upright. They also help us to rotate the spine and maintain good posture and the right amount of spinal curvature (neither too little or too much).

Spasms

When we strain or sprain our backs our muscles actually go into spasm. A muscle which is in spasm is in a contracted state.

There are two reasons why the back muscles will go into spasm, which are:

1. The muscles are trying to protect themselves from further strain by contracting very hard "spasming". Pretty much every back pain which goes beyond the regular slight ache, involves some degree of spasm. We tend to think of spasm in the severest sense whereby we're literally lying on the floor having difficulty breathing and ready to call for an ambulance. But there are also spams which are less intense, but the muscle is still spasming. As a rule of thumb whenever we strain or sprain a back muscle there will be some degree of spasm. But chances are that you won't notice this, usually someone else has to point it out to you, but it's there nonetheless.

2. Muscle spasm can come about as a consequence of an underlying problem with the spine, such as :

- Degenerative disc disease

- Herniated disc

- Spinal stenosis

- Facet joint osteoarthritis

Needless to say regular back relief exercises won't do much for these anatomical issues, which is why you should always consult with your doctor, if you are having either severe pain/lack of mobility issues or you are having a back problem for an extended period of time and no amount of rehabilitation appears to be helping!

Treating Back Pain with Remedial Exercises

So from a treatment point of view when we want to treat our aching backs, so long as it's just the muscles, ligaments and tendons and not an anatomical problem, we have to find a way of relaxing these spasming muscles and also work on balancing the musculature of the back and rebuilding the back muscles to some degree.

To do this we have to try out stretching exercises, which will help to relieve the tension in the muscles, we have to look at postural exercises and core strengthening exercises to rebalance the posture and we have to look at strengthening exercises, so as to rebuild the back muscles and prevent further back problems from occurring in the future.

Stretching to Relieve Back Pain

Look at the list above we can see that we have to work on the oblique's, the flexors and the extensors, if we want relieve from back pain. The process of relieving back pain is a several stage process but it begins with stretching.

The idea behind stretching is to gently loosen out the tension in the various muscle groups in the back. It is necessary to relax the muscle, which is in spasm and also the surrounding muscles groups, as in some way they are also probably contributing to your aching back.

Stretching Guidelines

- Wear loose fitting comfortable clothes

- Make sure you have enough room to stretch and have a mat or some kind of cushions which you can sit, stand a lie on so that the stretching session is comfortable

- Move into the stretch position slowly do not force

- Hold the stretched for 20 to 30 seconds

- Repeat 5 to 10 times per stretch

- You can stretch anytime of the day you like. Ideally both morning and evening is good. Although do bear in mind that the body will usually be stiffer first thing in the morning, so maybe be up and about for an hour or so before you conduct you're full morning stretching session.

It's a good idea to stretch in the morning, so as to limber up the body and it's also a good idea to stretch in the night so that the body is relaxed while going asleep. Especially when going to sleep, if you have a sore back it's a good idea to take whatever pain medication you have and do some light stretching, so that your back can relax. Often when we have a bad back, we have difficulty sleeping and we wake up feeling as stiff as a board. So muscle relaxing medication and light stretching prior to bedtime can really help if the pain is bad.

Stretching Exercises

Neck and Shoulders

Flexion Stretch – Chin to the Chest

To perform this exercise while either standing or sitting, simply bend your head forward and try and touch your chin of off your chest or at least until a stretch is felt on the back of your neck.

Lateral Flexion – From the Ear to the Shoulder

In this exercise begin by gently bending the neck to one side, as if you were trying to touch the shoulder with your ear. Continue until you feel a stretch on the side of the neck, and then try it out on the other side.

Trapezius and Shoulder Flexion – Shrug

This is a simple enough exercise. Simply lift up your shoulders as near as they can go to your ears, then let them drop down in a state of compete relaxation. Rest for a few seconds and then repeat. The idea is to squeeze your trapezius muscles at the top position, these are the two humps like muscles which sit upon the top of your shoulders. Squeezing and then letting go releases tension in the traps and the shoulders.

Back Stretching

Back Flexion Exercise

Iie on your back and with knees bent while your feet are in contact with the lower, reach forward with both hands and clasp under your knees and pull both knees to your chest while pulling your head forwards until you come into a balled up position.

Knee to Chest Stretch

Lying on your back with your knees bent and at the same time your heels are in contact with the floor, place both hands he bind one knee and bring it towards the chest.

Hip and Glute Stretch

Hip Stretch

This exercise is often called the happy baby pose because in this exercises you are going to lie on your back and pull your knees in towards your chest and then grab your feet and pull your hips as far s they go. By the time you start to get a good stretch on your hips you will look at a baby lying on their back and grabbing their feet!

Hip and Glute Activation

Hip and glute activation is also really important for most of us these days we are physically inactive most of the time. Because we spend so much of our time sitting at desks, siting in cars and trains and on bikes and siting on chairs and couches, our hips and glutes are tight, but also they are inactive. Often our glutes (ass muscles) are not active. On a physical level this will give the appearance of a small bottom and a funny walk, but also when the glutes are not doing their work the back is doing too much work. So a great way to prevent back pain is to activate the glutes and hams with the following exercises, which should be practiced on a daily basis. This exercise will get the glues and hams working and also it will give your lower back a nice stretch too!

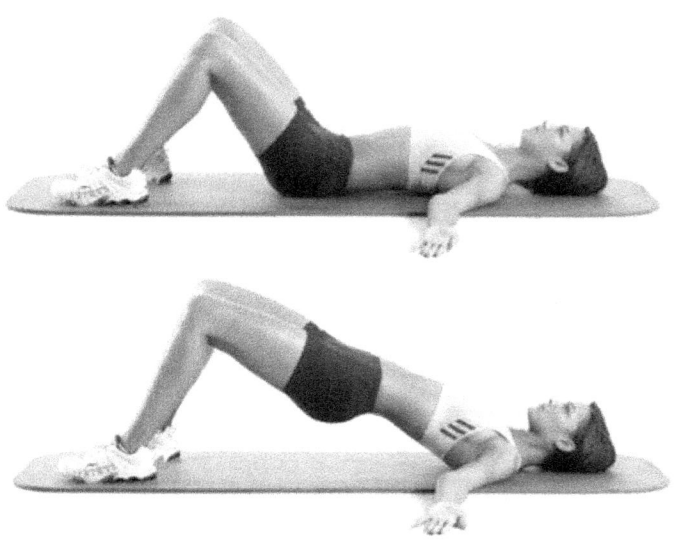

Picture courtesy of http://www.top.me/fitness

1. In a lying position, place your hands beside your head or beside your shoulders and with your feet pull them in as close a possible to your bottom, so that you are now lying on your back with your feet near your bottom.
2. Now while supporting your head with your hands push up with your legs so that your back arches, As it does so you will have to drive with your glutes and hamstrings and also you will feel a a stretch in your lower back. Your entire back will be arched to some degree and your hands will support your neck in the process.
3. Go up and then hold for a second and come down. Repeat ten times, take a 30 second break and then repeat again. Do three sets in total.

Piriformis Muscle Stretch

The piriformis muscles run through the buttock and can cause back or leg pain. In this exercise you are going to lie on your back and lift one leg upward and then grab the ankle with the opposite hand. So if you are lifting say your left leg up, then pull with your right arm and try and pull the ankle towards the right shoulder. Be careful to not put stress upon your knee, so hold your knee if need be and also pull with your knee but lead with your ankle.

An easier variation is too simple cross one leg over the other, so that say your left foot is just over your right knee and then with your right hand pull the knee towards the right shoulder, while making a point of not pulling the left hip up of off the floor. You will know if you are doing it correctly if you get a nice stretch in your buttocks. This exercise is a great way to loosen up the piriformis, which can help to relive back ache and also sciatica too!

Hamstring Stretching

Standing Hamstring Stretch

In this exercise you simply do the good old fashioned bending over from a standing position routine, whereby you stand and while keeping your legs either straight or nearly straight, you bend over and try to touch your toes. For many of us it might be difficult to get much past our knees, well don't worry about it, just try and stretch as fast forward as you can until you feel some resistance in your hamstrings. Once you feel the stretch just hold this position and after a few seconds chances are you will be able to go a little farther. Over a period of time you will come closer and closer to your toes!

If you have a lower back injury, you might be hardly able to bend at all, well once again just do what you can, even a slight movement forward will help over time to loosen things out.

Also, if you find that you cannot touch your toes, even after months of practice, chances are that you have tight calves!

Lying Hamstring Stretch

In this stretch begin by lying on your back, then bend one of your legs and pull it up of off the ground. Then reach out with both hands and grab this leg near the knees and pull on the knee while trying your best to keep your leg straight. You might feel a stretch in the hamstrings ounce your leg is a few inches of off the ground, well hold this position and after a few seconds try and go a little deeper and then hold it there for another fifteen to twenty seconds. Over time a stage will come when you can get your leg fully vertical and in some case it is even possible to bring the leg back further than 180 degree.

Calf Stretches

And let's not forget about calf stretches!

Just about everybody knows about bending forward and touching our toes but what about stretching our calves?

Often hamstring tightness will relate back to calf tightness and also a painful condition of the sole of the foot, which is known as plantar fasciitis. In plantar fasciitis, the tissue which runs between the heel of your foot and your toes becomes over tightened, which in turn can cause a lot of pain and discomfort when walking. However, it comes about as a consequence of over tightness in the calves and simply stretching the calf's over time will cure this condition!

Forward and Back Calf Stretch from a Seating Position

In this stretch you are going to point your toes forward and down. You will feel some tension on the top part of your foot. Then flip back the other way and this time bring your heel down while pulling your toes upwards, as if you wanted to pint your toes towards the sky., You will find that there is very little movement here because there is not much movement available in this joint but certainly you will feel a very distinct stretch in your calf muscle. Hold this for fifteen to twenty seconds and then flip back the other way and then repeat several times.

Calf Stretch from a Standing Position

In this variation you stand up and find yourself a wall. Then lift your toes upwards as high as they can go and press them against the wall. You can also do it from a sitting position by sitting and pressing your foot against a wall or office desk or whatever. Say you're at work and are sitting at your desk and the desk has some drawers, then while sitting press your toes against the drawers. So your heel should be on the floor a few inches away from the wall or drawers and your toes are pointing upwards and are pressed against the wall or drawers. Keep praising forward trying to bring your heel towards the wall or drawers, which is actually impossible (because there is not much movement in this joint and from a standing or sitting position, your calf is at a 45 degree angle already) but just do it until you feel a good stitch don then hold it there.

McKenzie Exercises for Slipped or Herniated Discs

We have been talking a lot about exercises for your back, stretching and so on and if you have a more serious back problem it can seem unbelievable to array out any of these exercises. However, if you have problems with your dics McKenzie exercises are a good place to start!

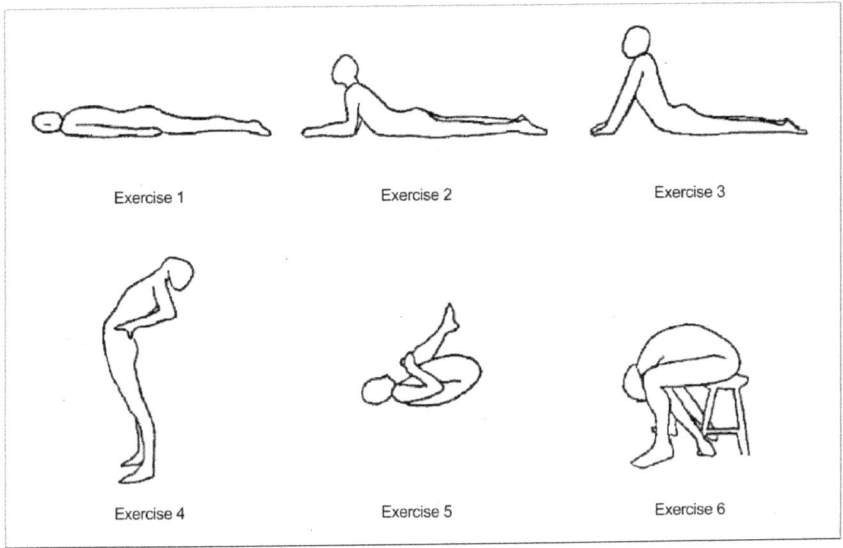

Exercise 1 Exercise 2 Exercise 3
Exercise 4 Exercise 5 Exercise 6

In this system of exercising you begin by lying face down for a about 30 seconds, and if you feel up to it then move into exercise two whereby you are propping yourself up on your elbows. Then bring yourself back down again and repeat. The idea with the McKenzie exercises isn't to run through all six exercises initially, but rather to rehab the lower back so as to help to realign the damaged disc.

You might find that you can only manage position one at first, if so then do this, but after a while try and move into position two, so along as pain and discomfort is moderate. After a while you can go into position three, which is a half cobra position (the cobra been a popular hatha yoga position).

Regarding exercise 5 and 6, with exercise 5 you will be laying on the floor and holding yourself in the foetal position, by pulling your knees up to your chest and in exercises six you will be in a sitting position and bending over and trying to reach the legs of a Stool.

Now looking over at exercise 4, this is probably the easiest exercise to perform. Here you simply stand and holding your lower back for support with your hands you stretch backwards until you can feel some tension in the lower back, hold for a few seconds and then return back to a vertical position.

The thing to bear in mind with these exercises is that they are all based on the premises of rehabbing a damaged disc in your lower back. When a disc is damaged in the lower back, it has a tendency to either expand outwards form its correct position or leak some of its synovial fluid. With these exercises the idea is to slowly help to realign the dice back into its correct position.

Secondly depending upon the type of disc problem you are having, some of these exercises will feel easier than others. As noted the standing exercise number 4 is probably the easiest, for many people performing exercise 3 will be much harder, while for most people exercise 5 will be the hardest. But you might find this reversed, it all depends upon how your back is. The golden rule with back problems is to begin with the least point of resistance and slowly work your way back towards health!

Fort a nice explanation video regarding getting started take a look at this video link here to a video which I found on You Tube.

Core Strengthening Exercises

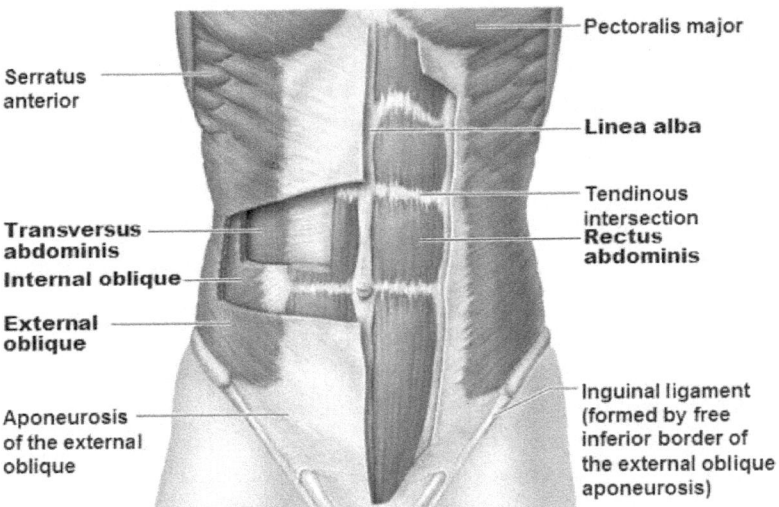

The muscles of our core are vitally important, if we want to maintain a healthy back, for when our core is strong we have a good posture and are largely free form postural imbalances, which usually kick of the back pain in the first place.

There are a wide variety of core exercises which you can practice, but the ones which follow are relatively easy keeping in mind that if you're reading this book, you probably have a bad back and cannot carry out some of these exercises without pain, so let's take a look at these easy one's.

Uddiyana Bandha

Uddiyana bandha (flying upwards) is actually a hatha yoga purification technique, but I am including it here because it also helps to strengthen our core muscles.

There are various approaches to carrying out Uddiyana bandha, personally I prefer a slow approach which is quite different from the way most people perform it. To perform Uddiyana bandha simply stand up and then crouch over slightly, while placing the palms of your hands on your thighs. Then breathe out and then when all the air is gone, suck in your abs muscles towards your back bone, as if a cord or thread where pulling in your navel. Feel the muscles contract hard, hold for a second and then let go and repeat again several more times. Take a deep breath and then repeat again for a another few times.

This is a little bit different from the way most practitioners practice it, as instead of going for a slow repetition cadence, they breath out very quickly and pull their abs in and out ten times in quick succession. You can try either approach, but I find that the fast approach will only work well for skinny people with very good ab control. If your abs are weak it will be difficult to perform this quickly and also if you have a flabby belly, the flab will make repaid repetitions difficult. I always recommend strictness of technique over speed. Try and feel the abs really working. But either way if you practice this exercise regularly, you will see a great improvement in the strengthens of you core. It not only strengthens the abs, but also it strengthens all of the muscles within the core region. Also it's great for intestinal health and to also helps to prevent or improve diabetes, because it stimulates the pancreas as well!

Cat and Cow

The cat and cow is basically a yoga exercise which has become popularised thanks to Pilates and consists of the following two movements.

For the cat position:

1. Begin by sitting on all fours on a mat or mattress, keeping your arms and legs shoulder width apart.

2. Squeeze your abs a little bit so they are strained and your back is straight.

3. Breathe in and when you breathe out, pull your abdominal muscles up while you arch your back up in the air like a cat, while your head and bottom are turned downwards towards the floor.

The Cow:

1. From the cat pose shift now by dropping your back down into a slightly curved position with your bottom and shoulders facing upwards.

2. Drop your lower lumbar region of your back down while maintaining a steady position with your bottom and keep with your shoulders and head up and facing forward. You will feel a stretch in your lumbar region of your back when you do this exercise.

The Plank

The plank is a famous core strengthening exercise and basically it consist of getting down on your hands and knees with your legs shoulder width apart and then pressing your body up into the same position as if you were going to do a push up, but instead of doing pushes you simply stay there for at least 20 seconds and if you can last 30 seconds than that's even better.

This can be a tough exercise especially if you have back pain, but if you stick with it over time it will really help to make the muscles of your core tight and strong. Initially it's ok to just stay in position for a few seconds but over a period of time slowly increases until you can hold this position for about 30 seconds.

Back Strengthening Exercises

An Important part of rehabbing our backs, involves strengthening our backs and a good place to start is with the McKenzie exercises above. Now you don't have to follow the protocol itself, but exercises number 2, 3 and 4 are a good starting point for developing some back strength.

Moving on from this you can always try out the hatha yoga exercises in the next section. In particular Bhujangasana (Cobra), Adho mukha śvānāsana (downward-facing dog Pose), ARDHA MATSYENDRASANA (Half Spinal Twist Pose) are all good exercises for strenethgnin your back muscles, you can find them in the next chapter.

Resistance Exercises

Other exercises which can be considered are resistance exercises such **as side bends**, whereby you begin by taking a book and holding it in your hand and then standing straight you bend to one side until you feel a slight stretch, then repeat 10 times each side. So hold a book in your right hand and turn leftwards ten times, with a book in your hands, and then repeat for 10 repetitions on your right hand side. After a while you can take up a dumbbell and do these exercises. This exercise works the serratus and the oblique's, which run along the side of our torso and help to stabilize the body and improve posture. You know this exercise is working when you feel a good stretch on the side opposite to the side which is holding a book.

Another good weight resistance exercise is single arm **dumbbell rows,** which can be carried out with a book at first and after a while you can start using a dumbbell. In this exercise you find a bench and with your left hand you support your body while your left knee rests on the bench. Meanwhile your right leg is straight. Now you take the book or dumbbell and lift it from the floor starting with the book or the dumbbell been just over hip height and then pull it up and back towards the wing like muscles in your back which are known as lattissimus dorsi muscles. If you are doing this exercise correctly your body should form a triangle shape, with one knee, one foot and your head making the three points of the triangle and your back maintaining a straight position throughout. This is a great exercise for developing these outer back muscles.

If you have access to a gym, you can try out the **lat pull-down machines,** of which there are quite a few variations available in most commercial gyms. Also another great exercise, which you can try in the gym is the **deadlift**. In deadlifting we begin by taking a bar and adding some weights, then sit down onto our haunches grab the weight and stand up. It's actually quite a technical exercise and you can hurt yourself if you're not careful so ask an instructor on how to perform this exercise. Of course you can always do a free form version of this exercise at home. Take a broom or a stick and from a standing position crouch down until you're on your hunkers and then keeping your back straight, stand up and keeping your back fairly straight, making sure at the completion of this exercise that your shoulders are pulled back slightly. Then repeat about 10 to 20 times, this will make one set, take a one minute break and repeat two more sets.

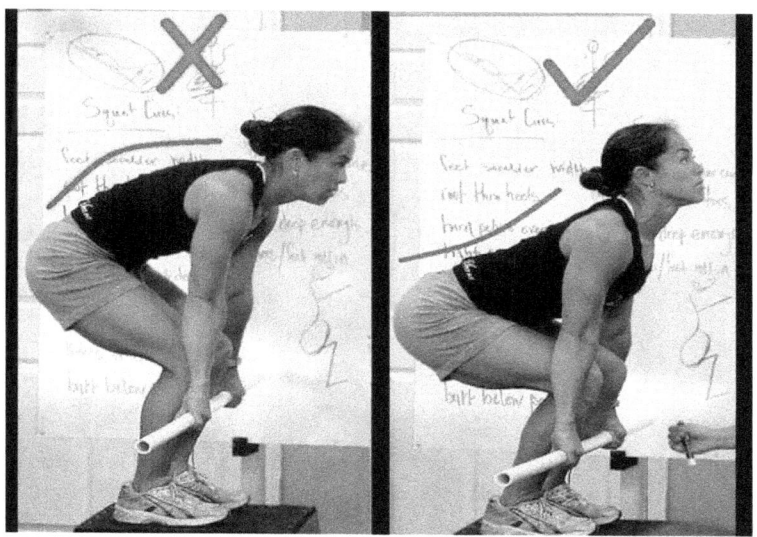

Deadlifting Picture courtesy of Pinterest user: sarahakaschmidy

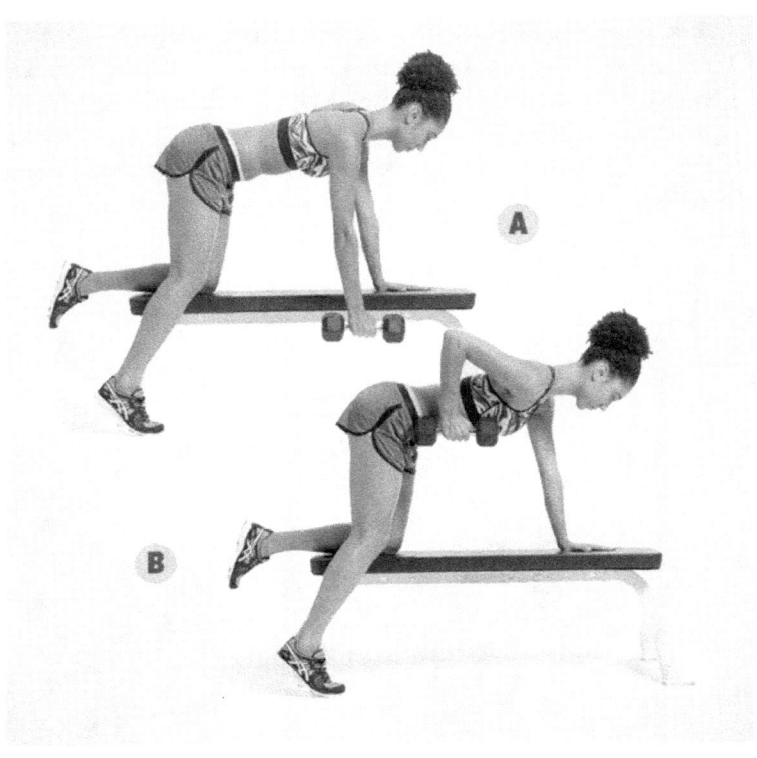

Single Arm Dumbbell Row Picture courtesy of Women's health Magazine on Pinterest

Even if you don't attend a gym, the deadlift is a great exercise for its works the entire posterior chain developing the muscles of the legs, back, rear arms, rear shoulders and traps. If you do this exercise without any weights, it will nicely tone your back and leg muscles and greatly improve your posture. If you perform it with weights, you will develop a thick muscular back, but it's potentially dangerous and you need to learn from a qualified instructor, how to do the deadlift and spend a few months practicing it once a week to get good at it!

Making Sense out of Remedial Back Exercises – Where to Start

In this chapter we have covered a lot of ground on the subject of remedial exercises for back health, but what's the best way to get a start with all of this?

Well this is the million dollar question, for it all depends upon where you're at with your back pain. If your back pain is not very intense and is just a dull chronic pain, then you can tackle stretching, core exercises, remedial exercises and strength building exercises form the get go. However, if your back is in an acute state, whereby you can hardly move then you have to use your common sense regarding where you want to begin. If you're presently in a lot of pain and having difficult with mobility, a good place to start is light stretching exercise, acupressure and some myosfascial release exercises. The other more extreme stretching and strength based exercises can all follow, when you have made considerable improvement with your back pain.

The key is to start gently and work your way through your back pain. Rehabbing first and then as things improve working on balancing and strengthening your back, so as to prehab it. In the next chapter, we shall look at hath yoga poses so once again these are really to be used when you have recovered from acute pain and are on the way back to back health and you are looking for prehabbing as much as rehabbing. But the final chapter on herbal teas is a really good place to begin with, if you are suffering from acute back ache for the various herbal tea's can provide pain relief, anti-inflammatory properties and healing properties in some cases.

What we have to remember when dealing with acute back pain is that the first thing which we have to do is make ourselves comfortable, for only when we start to relax the muscles and reduce the pain can the body begin the process of healing. The next stage is to start rebalancing and finally rebuilding the back muscles.

So always begin with an end in mind. So if, for example, you have just pulled your back and are in acute pain, start by taking herbal teas and using external rubs plus allopathic pain fillers/anti-inflammatory. Try and rest the muscles and if you have just pulled a muscle you can use ice to reduce inflammation, but within 24 hours the body will have filled the area with blood in an effort to mend the damage. So by this stage ice should not be used, rather heat should be used so as to improve the blood circulation in the damaged area. So you might use ice initially, but then after a few hours after the pull use eucalyptus rub, which is hot. You use ice initially to reduce the swelling, but after a few hours you use heat to warm up the region. Then slowly start moving this body part and other body parts so as to stimulate a healing response.

Try to make concerted effort to make yourself comfortable before sleep which will probably involve some light stretching, a warm external rub with some pain relieving cream, an allopathic pain killer, and some herbal pain relieving tea and then sleep.

After a few days as life starts to come back to the affected area, increase movement and consider adding in things like a light walk or possible a light stair climb, so as to gently stimulate the back. After another few days or week or two, as the acute pain gives way to a chronic pain, work at more core balancing and advanced stretching exercises. After a while try and pick up on where there are imbalances, in your back and add in other exercises, such as hatha yoga exercises and resistance exercises so as to rebalance the back, finish off the rehab and progress with the prehab so as to prevent further back injuries form taking place.

Chapter Six – Hatha Yoga

Hatha yoga of one of the six branches of yoga. The word yoga means to unite and the advanced yogi will practice yoga physical health postures (hatha yoga), meditation (mantra yoga), spiritual devotion (bhakti yoga), wisdom (jana yoga), fulfilling one's duty (karma yoga) and higher spiritual meditation and mental training(raja yoga). Hatha yoga is the most famous branch, because it focuses upon rebalancing the physical body. In the process of doing this it helps the yogi to advance towards the goal of integration of body, mind and spirit, but for our needs we are just going to focus upon the physical therapeutic benefits of hatha yoga postures.

From the point of view of healing back pain, there are several distinct advantages with hatha yoga postures, which are:

- Pretty much most hatha yoga poses are based upon manipulation of the spine, so most hatha yoga poses (asanas) will help to work on balancing the back in some form or other.

- Regular hatha yoga practice will rebalance the muscles in the back and indeed the muscles which run along the entire posterior chain (muslces of the back, legs, rear arms, rear shoulders and neck). Since most bad back problems originate with postural imbalances, anything which helps to rebalance these muscle groups over time, will eventually help to prevent the reoccurrence of back ache. From this point of view hatha yoga postures can be seen as prehab (pre-habilitation as in a preventative).

- Hatha yoga posture will help to rehab (repair damage) as they will gently help to rebalance the various muscle groups and also they will help to tone up the musculature of the back, thus making the back more functional thus curing back ache!

- The emphasize on spinal movements and the improved flow of subtle pranic energy (prana is the Indian way of describing Qi (Chi) energy, a subtle energy which lies behind the effective functioning of all bodily activities). Hatha yoga will help spinal health as well and in some cases regular and careful practice can help to overcome physical deformities of the spine to some degree. For example, minor cases of spondylosis can sometimes be cured and herniated discs in the back, in some cases, can either be cured or greatly improved upon.

- Also because with hatha yoga we're not just carrying out a physical therapy, but rather we are moving subtle energy around the body, as a consequence of this hatha yoga has a strong simulating effect upon the nervous system and may help to relieve nerve pain, in some cases!

The thing with hath yoga is that there are many levels to hatha yoga, so we must be careful with how we approach hatha yoga. The atypical images of hath yoga usually shows a beautiful young woman in an athletic poise, but in reality hatha yoga is carried out by people of all ages and genders, so anybody either young or old can give it a try. However, the advanced postures are difficult and can even be dangerous sometimes, so you just can't jump in there and think that you can practice hath yoga, in the same way that you might take up a dance class!

Hatha yoga is an ancient system of physical rejuvenation and was designed carefully over many hundreds of years. The student begins with easy posies and over a period of months and years they work their way into the more difficult exercises. Like any endeavour there is a learning curve and like all physical exercises if you're foolish you will hurt yourself.

Also before beginning any exercise protocol you have e to evaluate yourself. Are you reasonably fit, are you over weight, how old are you, what physical infirmities do you have, do you have any health problems like high blood pressure for instance?

According to how you answer these questions you can approach hatha yoga. For example some people are really inflexible, while others can hop into a difficult poise with relative ease. In summary start slow and easily and work up to the more difficult poses and be sensible.

Also another important consideration, not only with hatha yoga but with all eastern physical exercises, is that hatha yoga is not a fitness class (although some people teach it as if it were), rather it's a system of physical reintegration, so it's not about "going for the burn" or knocking out endless reps, rather it's about doing the exercises slowly and deeply and getting into the exercises. With hatha yoga, when you start getting into the exercises you will notice your breathing deepen and your mind settle down and become more relaxed, this is the way it should be because not only are you stretching and toning the muscles, but rather you are also moving subtle pranic energy currents around the body, thus balancing the body, mind and spirit. If you just focus on the psychical you will get a workout, but if you go with the flow and stop worrying about reps and instead try to get into the posture and feel it work, you will be surprised at how good you will feel after it!

Finally what follows are all easy postures, but if you want to take it to the next level there's lots of information online regarding yoga postures or you can join a yoga class in your local area. But one thing to remember, prior to joining a yoga class do check it out and make sure that they are emphasizing the feel of the exercises, it should not be like a yoga version of a Zumba class!

Two Forward bending Poises

What follows are two great forward bending poses, which can do wonders for back health, but bear in mind that they can be detrimental for a person who has **DISC PROBLEMS WITH THEIR BACK**. You can always try to out gently and see how you feel, but as a rule of thumb neither exercise should be practiced by anyone with disc problems!

Uttanasana (Intense Forward-Bending Pose)

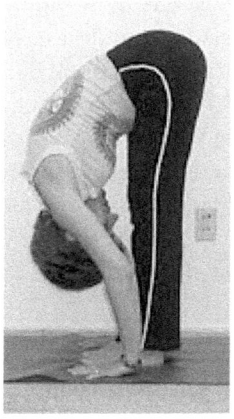

Picture courtesy of wikepedia

In this pose you simply stand straight and bend over tyring to press your head against your legs and with you hands, slowly pull yourself down so that ideally your hands can touch the soles of your feet.

Hatah yogi's atypically hold this posture for 2 or 3 minutes, the benefit been a good stretch on the hamstirngs and also it gives the entire spine a stretch.

However, for someone starting out, especially for a person with back pain, it's fine to go as deep as feels easy for you. Initially you might only be able to reach your knees with your hands. Well if this is all you can do then fine. You can always release, stand up again and then try to stretch again and then repeat several times as you loosen out until you feel that this is proabably as good as you will get. Then hold this position while gently pushing forward, you will find after a minute or so that you end up deepening your stretch and this is the key to hatha yoga exercises. It can be a good idea to repeat a few repeititons intitially just to limber up and get into the pose, but once you get into the pose don't stop and start, rather hold for a minute or two and slowly go a little deeper. While today you might be lucky, if you reach your knees with your hands and your head goes nowhere near your legs, after a few weeks you will be beale to reach your ankles with your hands!

Also it's not a race, so just do the best you can, afterall if you have damage to your back, the goal is to stretch and sterenghten your back so use this exercise remedially and don't try to cpmpete with anyone!

Pashchimottanasana (Seated Forward Bend)

Picture courtesy of wikepedia

Seated forward bend is the seating version of the previous exercise intense forward bending pose and if you are having a lot of mobility issues, with your back this might be the better exercise for you.

The basic instructions are the same as in bend forward as much as you can and place your head on your legs while pulling your body towards you toes with your fingers. Once again just do the best you can and focus on getting a deep stretch with the aim of pushing a little every day, this way your mobility will improve quickly and once again realise that due to back injury, you may not be able to reach your toes which is ok, what's more important is the remedial and prehab effects of stretching the back and toning the muscles in the back and also relaxing the hamstrings.

From a back health point of view both if these exercises release the hamstrings which in turn will help to release pressure on both the calf muscles and the lower back. Often back problems relate back to tightness in the calf's and hamstrings. When we stretch our hamstrings, it relaxes our calves and the soles of our feet and lower back as well, so hamstring stretches are always a good idea.

Earlier I me motioned that the entire back portion of the body is referred do as the posterior chain and this is very relevant, for like a chain every muscle group and joint in this chain pulls on each other, so often a small imbalance will throw out your back. If you want a healthy back then work on balancing out the various muscle groups, ligaments and tendons in your posterior chain.

Also as an aside both of these exercises will increase blood flow into the lower intestines and pancreas thus helping to boost digestion and blood sugar control!

Bhujangasana (Cobra)

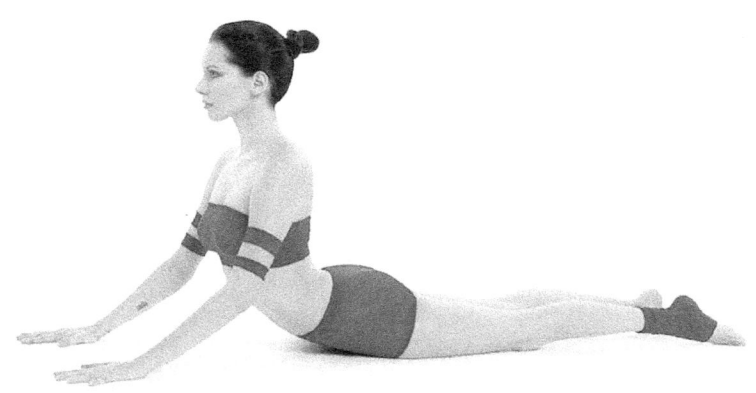

Picture courtesy of wikipedia user Kennguru

alexey baykov yogashaktipat.com yoga.shaktipat@gmail..com

The cobra is a famous hatha yoga pose and it's pretty obvious as to where the name comes from, because in this pose you raise yourself up as if you were a king cobra snake!

To practice it is fairly simple, you lie on the floor with hands parallel to your face, just like in downward dog, but instead of raising your bottom in the air you push your upper torso up with your arms. The idea is to push until your arms are fully extended and you feel a good stretch in the lower back. The key to getting the stretch in the lower back is to push yourself up as high as you can go. Once there hold this posture and make a point of keeping your eyes looking straight ahead, don't arch your neck. If you are doing it correctly you should feel a nice feeling of strain and tension through your arms, shoulders and back and in particular the lower back.

Hold this position for several breaths, then release and let your body lie down and then repeat a couple more times.

This is a great exercise both for upper body strength and also for stretching and releasing tension in the lower back. Also in its peak position it helps to balance the upper rose, neck and shoulders thus improving posture as well!

Adho mukha śvānāsana (downward-facing dog Pose)

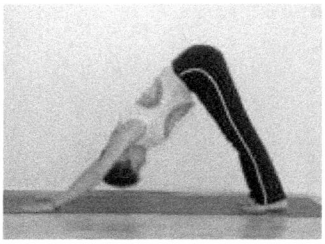

Picture courtesy of wikipedia

Downward facing dog is an alround body builder. It particualry developes the trapezius muscles of the pper back, the latissimus dorsi (outer back muscles), the back of the arms (tricpes), the bottom (gluteus maximus) and the back of the thighs (hamstrings). It also has a secondary effect on the mid back (rhomboids), the primary shoulder tendons (rotator cuff), the front and side shoulder msucles (anterior and medial deltoids), the rear shoulder muslces (posterior deltoids) the muscles of the lower side of the body (serratus), and the calf muscles (soleus and gastrocnemius).

Now where this exerise helps the rehab and prehab of back pain is because it tones up all the muscles of the posterior chain and it also tighten sthe core muscles of the midsection. It tighterns up the abdomen and the lower back muscles and the side muscles (the serratus), which make the physicque more stable and grounded thus helaing old injuries and preventing new ones from taking place.

To perfrom this exercise simply lie down with your face toughicng the floor and your hands palm downwards parallel to your face. Now lift your bottom and hips up from the floor while pushing up both with the heels of your feet and your hands pushing upwards so that your body will now resemble a rof with fet and hands at oppsite ends and your bottom at the peak postion.

Now ideally you should stay in this position for between 20 to 25 breaths, which could be very taxing at the early stages. More importabtly when in this peak position try to fiocus on breahting in and out steadily and feeling the energy movemetn with the body. Try and feel the exercises, feel your breaht, feel the energy flow and the tension in the muscles. If you can only stay in this possition for a few breahts then fine you will increase over time!

Bālāsana (Child's Resting Pose)

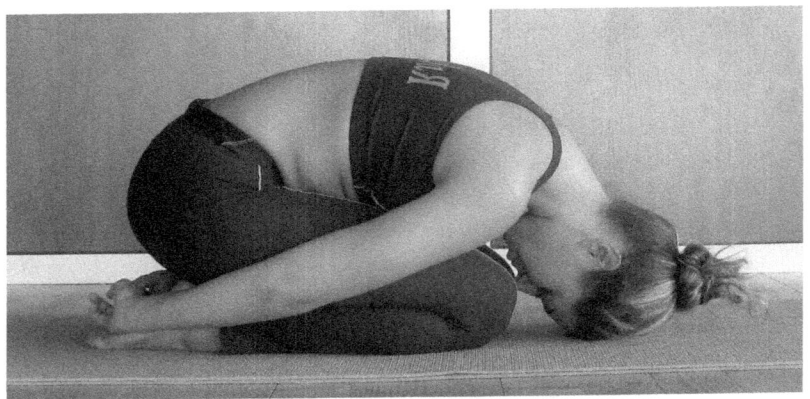

Picture courtesy of wikipedia

After performing downward facing dog the relaxed poise to follow straight afterwards is the child's resting pose. It's failry straight forward to oerform. Simply sit down on your knees and let your torso lay down on your thighs and your head on the floor or as near to the floor as possibel. Also you have to let your amrs droop and relax while holding your hands over your heels.

Now for many of us this is a tough pose to perfrom correctly as we tend to be so stiff that it's difficult to reach the floor with our heads and even our torso's get stuck halfway down with our shoulders and heads been way of the floor. However, with practice the position will become easier to perfrom. The key is absolute relaxation of the back muscles and this is also why this exercise combines so well with downward dog because we have just drilled our back muscles and now we give them complete rest. Try and feel the muslces of your mid back and simply let them stretch and relax, as they do so your torso and head will dropp down.

This exercise is a relaly great way to take stress out of your back and also its really good for spinal health and general rest and relaxation!

ARDHA MATSYENDRASANA (Half Spinal Twist Pose)

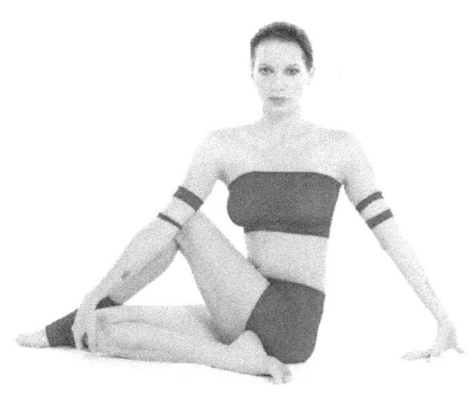

Picture courtesy of wikipedia user Kenngurualexey baykov yogashaktipat.com yoga.shaktipat@gmail..com

This is a great poise for working on stretching the latsissimus dorsi muslces of the back (the outer back muscles). Also it creates a stretch from the hips right through the width of the back and right up into the beck which gives the entire back area a good stretch. In particualr while stretching the nerves which run along the spine are simualted with fresh blood and so too are the ligaments and tendons. This exercise is good for both rehabd and prehab and if practised regulary it will go a long way towards ensuring back health.

It's a little ticky to get it right at ifrst as the posie feels cotner intuitive. Basicalu you are going to sit with your left leg crossed over your folded right knee and then holding the right knee with your right hand while reaching around almost towafrds your back with your left hand and then pulling the spine into a gentle twist. Hold the position until you feel a good stretch and take a few breahs. Release and then do again three more times. Then swap over this time you will be turning your torso to the right hand side and placing your reight leg over your folded left knee, repeat four times in total!

One foot is placed flat on the floor outside the opposite leg and torso twists toward the top leg. The bottom leg may be bent with the foot outside the opposite hip, or extended with toes vertical. The arms help leverage the torso into the twist and may be bound (Baddha Ardha Matsyendrasana) in a number of configurations by clutching either feet or opposite hands.

Chapter Seven - Herbal Remedies for Back Pain

If you have read any of my other books then chances are that you came across some information relating back to herbal remedies. My interest in herbal remedies kicked off when I was training to become a Traditional Chinese Medical (TCM) practitioner. I was quite amazed at the sheer effectiveness of these herbal remedies and over the years I have checked out quite a few herbs and always to my surprise there are so many natural remedies in easy access of everyone, but we just don't realize that these herbs can help. So give them a try you might be surprised at just how much pain relief you get!

Herbal Teas for Back Pain Relief

Tumeric

Turmeric is a famous Indian spice which has a beautiful bright yellow color and which is known for its food enhancing qualities, but it also makes for a real healthy tea!

Turmeric is high in cucumin, which is high in anti-inflammatory properties. It can also be used as a rub for external use!

Valerian Root

Valerian root when turned into a tea is a fantastic sleep aid. It reduces pain and helps one to get asleep quickly and stay asleep. For anyone who has difficulty sleeping with back pain a cup of valerian tea is worth trying out prior to bed time!

Eucommia

Encomia are ancient Chinese herbs which was popular for its ability to reduce pain in aching joints and also for back pain relief. This herb reduces pain and also helps to heal soft tissue damage!

White Willow Bark

White willow bark is a strong pain reliever, and appears to be high in aspirin like compounds. It works well for both acute and chronic back aches!

Devils Claw

Devils claw is well known for its ability to reduce pain and swelling in osteoarthritis patients. It is high in anti-inflammatory properties and works well on both back and neck pain also.

Black Cohosh

Black cohosh works particular well on muscle spasms and since back pain consists mostly of muscle spasms this is a great way to reduce not only the achiness but also the tension in the back muscles thus paving the way towards rehabilitation of the back musculature.

Kava Kava

Kava Kava is quite famous for its anti-depressant like properties but is also good for pain relief. It's a strong relaxant and works well along with other herbs at relaxing the back and acting as a natural sedative which is especially good before going to sleep with a sore back!

How to Make Herbal Tea

Kava Herbal tea is surpassingly easy to prepare just follow these instructions:

1. Take out the root or herb which you want to use.
2. Place it in 300ml of alter per cup.
3. Boil the water.
4. Leave to simmer for 10 minutes.
5. Strain and serve.

Some of these herbal teas taste better than others so it's always a good idea to experiment. Also you can try combining different herbs which may enhance taste and certainly it will enhance the effectiveness of the herbs!

Free Gift

Grab Free Books!!!!!!!!

As a way of saying thank you for downloading this book I would like to give you two free books, which are available exclusively for my readers. The free book "Juicing for Health – 35 Juicing Recipes for Everyday Health Problems", is packed full of useful healthy juice recipes and Success Hacks - 31 Mind-Set Hacks to Increase Productivity and Career Success, is packed full of helpful mind hacks for developing a more dynamic and enjoyable lifestyle!

Please click on the link to receive your gift.